Hush: A Book of Bedtime Contemplations

"The science is in: There's practically no element of our lives that's not improved by getting adequate sleep. *Hush* draws on the latest sleep science to take us deeper, exploring sleep's spiritual, sacred, and transformative dimensions and guiding us toward the deep, restorative sleep our bodies and our souls need."

–Arianna Huffington, President and Editor-in-Chief of The Huffington Post Media Group

"These 100 gems by one of the leading experts on sleep will change your relationship with what you do with one-third of your life! Sometimes poetic, sometimes paradoxical, often surprising, your understanding of sleep and dreams will be enriched and your ability to 'descend gradually into sleep like the sun into the sea' will be enhanced."

–David Feinstein, PhD, Co-director of Innersource

"Dr. Rubin Naiman challenges us to reconsider what night consciousness may hold for us. In so doing, he helps all of us to sleep better."

–Victoria Maizes, MD, Executive Director, University of Arizona Center for Integrative Medicine

"Finally, a sleep-supportive book that speaks to the spirit as well as the mind. These nonaddictive prescriptions provide an excellent prelude to sleep for both individuals and couples. I highly recommend this work to those who struggle with sleep as well as those who want to deepen their experience of sleep and dreams."

–Terry Real, founder of Relational Life Institute

"Dr. Rubin Naiman has long been recognized as a global leader in integrative approaches to sleep and dreams. In *Hush,* he offers us is a unique, thoughtful, and poetic work that takes a huge step toward healing the rift between the spirit and science of sleep. I read several nuggets last night before bed and had my best night's sleep in ages!"

–Emerson Wickwire, PhD, ABPP, CBSM, Director, Insomnia Program, University of Maryland

"I was very impressed with Dr. Naiman's book, especially so because there is so little written about the emotional and spiritual factors causing insomnia and poor sleep. Dr. Naiman is commended for providing a very straightforward way for insomnia patients to seek what amounts to a very natural healing path for sleepless nights."

–Barry Krakow, MD, Medical Director of Maimonides Sleep Arts & Sciences

"Rubin Naiman has been one of our wisest sleep and dream pioneers and teachers for decades. With *Hush,* Dr. Naiman takes his accumulated wisdom from science, psychology, spirituality and culture and applies it with poetic vision and deep love and gentleness to all issues regarding sleeping and dreaming. This is a deceptively simple and beautifully composed book that not only offers wise and gentle meditations for improving sleep and dream life it also integrates science and spirituality and steers us all toward a new and deep valuing of sleeping and dreaming.

–Edward Tick, PhD, Co-founder and Executive Director of Soldier's Heart

"The best prescription for sleepless patients."

–Randy Horwitz, MD, PhD, Medical Director of the Arizona Center for Integrative Medicine

Hush

A Book of Bedtime Contemplations

Rubin Naiman PhD

ISBN: 0615979424
ISBN 13: 9780615979427
Library of Congress Control Number: 2014904436
NewMoon Media, Tucson, AZ

For Hugh Prather

Acknowledgements

My heartfelt gratitude is extended to Stefanie Marlis and Erin Lamb for their invaluable editorial and emotional support. Additional thanks go to Terry Real, Amy Weintraub, David Hochner, and Suzie Massey for their kind and helpful feedback. I am deeply grateful to Andrew Weil, Victoria Maizes, Randy Horwitz, and Tieraona Low Dog at the University of Arizona Center for Integrative Medicine for providing me with a nurturing academic environment to evolve my work. And, as always, I am thankful to my patients who have taught me most of what I know about sleep and dreams.

Introduction

It's noisy out there. Sometimes it feels like there are wild and wounded things prowling about the night. And it can get pretty noisy in here, as well. An unsettling and relentless din echoes around our homes and hearts, disrupting our precious sleep.

Too often, we reflexively respond to all this noise by shouting right back at it. We grow frustrated, argue and plead with it. We strategize obsessively about controlling it. And we eventually declare war against it, issuing preemptive strikes with alcohol or marijuana or escalating nightly rounds of sleeping pills.

Although sleep science has significantly advanced our understanding of sleep, it has endorsed the use of dubious medications to manage sleeplessness. So-called sleeping pills essentially produce a kind of chemical white noise in the brain that doesn't actually quiet the din. It just temporarily dampens our ability to hear it.

Sleep science has, indeed, taught us much about sleep -- but not enough about the sleeper. Authentic sleep can't be reduced to squiggly EEG tracings and the complex cascade of bodily humors. Such an objective understanding is necessary but largely insufficient because it disregards the personal, subjective experience of the sleeper. This experience is best understood not through scientific but rather through personal investigation. The first step in such investigation is reclaiming responsibility for our sleep.

Over the past half century, sleep has been abducted from its natural home in our hearts and minds and has become exceedingly medicalized. We've been encouraged to view sleep as a strictly scientific and mechanistic phenomenon shrouded in medical complexities -- a perspective that significantly limits our personal access to it. The pharmaceutical industry has, in turn, emerged as the gatekeeper of sleep, strongly biasing the delivery of related information, research, and services.

Just as the natural childbirth movement arose to counter the medicalization of pregnancy and childbirth, we are in dire need of a natural sleep movement to counter the appropriation of sleep by the healthcare industry. We must actively reclaim sleep and reaffirm our personal authority over and responsibility for our own sleep. Doing so calls for a transformative shift in both cultural and individual attitudes.

Our challenge is to appreciate the physiological mechanisms of sleep without sacrificing its essential transcendent qualities. Because we can never fully understand sleep as an intellectual concept, we must learn to be comfortable with its mystery.

To fully "get" sleep -- that is, to both understand and obtain it -- we must be willing to let go of the preconceived notions we have about it. We must learn to approach it mindfully with patience, humility, and a willingness to learn directly from it. We must be willing to befriend and dialog with our own sleep in a new way.

Something serene and ineffable sweeps through the deep currents of night just beneath the din of the waking world. Sleep is inherently and profoundly peaceful -- so peaceful that most of us have absolutely no frame of reference for perceiving, let alone languaging it. The one aspect of sleep, however, that is most regularly accessible to us all is dreaming.

"A dream may lead us deeper into the secrets of nature than a hundred concerted experiments," wrote Ralph Waldo Emerson. Willingness to learn from sleep means keeping our hearts open to dreaming. It means cultivating receptivity to our nightly dreams, learning to access and remember them, and intentionally integrating their transcendent and spiritual perspectives into our waking lives.

Hush was born of an integration of sleep science and spirituality. It was written to complement effective behavioral sleep medicine approaches with more traditional sacred views of sleep and dreams. *Hush's* "prescriptions" are, therefore, meant to speak to the heart as well as the mind. They are not intended to provoke deep analysis but to invoke deep sleep.

Hush is not so much a book of sleep tips but one of sleep transformation. Although our activities can certainly hinder or promote sleep, it's important to remain cognizant of the fact that sleep itself is a state of mind, not an activity. Hugh Prather's sagacious advice is germane here: *Make your state of mind more important than what you are doing.*

The passages in *Hush* are intended to be gently contemplated. Consider reading one or more each night at bedtime. One can proceed sequentially through the book or just open it to a page at random.

Passage through the gateway of sleep requires a shift in consciousness. Whether we access it intentionally or just crash into it out of sheer exhaustion, sleep calls for a relinquishment of our ordinary waking ways of being. Mindfully entering the theater of sleep is much like entering a movie theater. We instinctively hush.

Rubin Naiman
March 2014
Tucson, Arizona

We don't get sleep because we don't 'get' sleep.

Our definitions of sleep are largely negative. That is, they tell us what sleep is *not*. In the same way we naively think of health as the absence of disease, we think of sleep as the absence of waking or the absence of consciousness. Scientifically, sleep is defined as non-REM -- it's not dreaming. Knowing what sleep is *not* does not tell us what it *is*. But "getting" that we don't know what it is, "getting" that it is a mystery is an essential step toward getting sleep.

∽ 2 ∾

Chronic sleeplessness is a symptom of our addiction to waking.

We live in a world that views waking consciousness as the quintessential human experience. Being awake is considered synonymous with being truly alive. When we're challenged with problems, including sleeplessness, we reflexively engage our waking mind to solve them. Sleeplessness, however, is not an ordinary problem because it commonly stems from our compulsive reliance on waking. We simply can't engage our waking mind to help us disengage from waking.

∽ 3 ∽

Going to bed with the same waking mindset we sported all day is like sleeping in our clothes.

Though most of us routinely change our clothes before bed, few of us effectively change our minds. We unthinkingly smuggle daytime waking ways of being into night's domain of sleep and dreams. Waking life is driven primarily by intention while night consciousness is primarily informed by receptivity. We know how to change our minds. We do it all the time. We simply need to remember and be willing to do so at bedtime.

〜 4 〜

Dreams are the mythic backstory
of our daily lives.

How do we turn the page at the end of each day? The essence of our everyday life stories is too easily obscured by the excessive detail stirred into them. We get distracted by the mundane and lose sight of what is truly sacred -- the challenging, adventurous, and mythic aspects of our lives. Our deeper Self cannot digest ordinary life until it's broken down into its molecular mythical components during dreaming. Dreams reveal the true story concealed behind "the real world" -- the story to be recorded in the book of our lives.

ᦂ 5 ᦁ

Darkness is the best sleep medicine.

If God or angels or extraterrestrials were indeed monitoring us from above, the most profound change they would have witnessed on this planet since its creation is the pernicious illumination of our nights. Satellite images taken of the planet at night reveal that it is glowing brighter with each passing year. Overexposed to light at night, many of us unknowingly suffer from a darkness deficiency. Darkness is not just the absence of light; it's also a kind of nourishment -- a bittersweet chocolate for the soul. It's best to sleep in total darkness.

6

Sleep is so much more than a servant of waking life; it's a rich and direct experience of life itself.

There is no question that sleep supports a healthy waking life in numerous ways. It restores our energy, promotes immunity, facilitates learning and memory, improves performance, enhances our appearance, and much more. But sleep is not simply a means to these ends. If we view sleep as being solely utilitarian, we fail to recognize its inherent deeper value and joy.

7

Poor sleep does not usually stem from insufficient sleepiness but from excessive wakefulness.

Whether we feel it or not, most of us are sufficiently sleepy at bedtime. This sleepiness, however, is readily veiled by wakefulness trespassing into our nights. Excessive wakefulness, also known as hyperarousal, results from a body and mind in chronic overdrive -- the psychophysiological equivalent of habitually exceeding the speed limit. Obscured against the backdrop of waking life, hyperarousal is most evident and unsettling in the dark and quiet of night. It calls for a gentle but persistent effort to slow down.

8

**From the perspective of waking,
falling asleep is an accident.**

Sleep is the slippery, downhill side of the day. We cannot intentionally go there. We can only slip, slide or fall into it. We slip out of waking and we fall -- which is suggestive of an accident -- asleep. Evening rest and relaxation make us accident-prone.

9

We view dreams the way we view stars: they are magnificent but far too distant to be of any relevance to our lives.

Because we live in a world where dreaming is so utterly misconstrued and widely dismissed, we fail to recognize the critical role it plays in our well being, happiness and spirituality. Despite its distance, the night sky is universally acknowledged for its natural grandeur -- for its romantic, artistic, poetic, and, of course, spiritual qualities. Could it be that our dreams, which are so much closer in, offer us something quite similar?

∽ 10 ∽

We cannot heal our relationship with sleep and dreams without first healing our relationship with night.

Hypnos, the Greek god of sleep, was the son of Nyx, the mighty goddess of night. Sleep, then, is the child of night. Night provides respite for our senses, facilitates the release of melatonin, and encourages deep sleep and dreams. Unfortunately, we commonly confuse night's literal darkness with the metaphor of darkness or evil. It's perfectly safe to surrender to night. Her darkness is a healing retreat, a carbon filter for the soul.

＄ | | ＄

Thinking of sleep as unconsciousness raises the risk of confusing it with the knockout of substances and sleeping pills.

Sedating substances and medications induce a chemical knockout -- a kind of unconsciousness. Even though sleep is commonly associated with a lack of awareness, it's a mistake to equate it with unconsciousness. Just because it looks like sleep doesn't mean that it is sleep. Sleep isn't unconsciousness; it's another kind of consciousness -- one that has never been effectively replicated through chemistry.

∽12∾

It's natural, common and normal to experience occasional sleeplessness.

Sometimes we just can't sleep. This can result from a stressful day, hormonal shifts and, yes, even the full moon. Occasional sleeplessness is not insomnia and does not usually require intervention. Worrying about occasional sleeplessness, however, can exacerbate it and, in fact, predispose us to insomnia. We can prevent this from happening by simply accepting and forgiving occasional sleeplessness as well as ourselves when it occurs.

༄ 13 ༄

Beyond all the complexities associated with it, falling asleep is an act of faith.

If we are to surrender to the mystery of sleep -- if we are to check out and relinquish oversight and control -- we need some sense of what will be watching over us, our families and all that is dear to us. Because falling asleep requires that we extend trust or faith to something greater than ourselves, it raises deeply spiritual questions. The extent of our willingness to surrender to sleep is the measure of this faith. The process of falling asleep, then, can be best understood as a personal spiritual practice.

ᴄᴏ | 4 ᴄᴏ

Dreaming is not optional; it's an essential part of good sleep and healthy waking.

Dreaming is critical for learning and memory. Dreams also play a key role in the regulation of our feelings and moods and in the psychological assimilation of daily life experiences. Dreaming provides an essential poetic cushion for our sharply literal lives. It serves as a palpable nightly reminder that the world is so much bigger than it appears to be by day. In dreams we are privy to a much grander conversation.

ᔥ 15 ᔦ

Our nightstands are a clear reflection of our stance toward night.

Our nightstands are an expression of our prevailing operational beliefs about sleep -- our personal sleep stories. If sleep is a nightly get-away, then the nightstand is the overnight bag we carry along with us. Are the items in and around our nightstands conducive to a surrender to sleep? Or do they tether us to the waking world with clocks, lamps, radios, computers, telephones or energy spiking foods and substances?

༄ 16 ༈

We are all always already asleep.

Sleep is our default -- a substrate of consciousness that
steadfastly resides beneath the din of ordinary waking life.
When we loosen our grip on waking, sleep naturally begins
to seep through. Sometimes it wafts into waking as a gracious
moment of inexplicable serenity. Close your eyes for a few
seconds and gently allow your awareness to turn inward
without any specific intention. Can you sense that part of
yourself that dwells in sleep right now?

ༀ 17 ༀ

When sleep becomes an issue, it is typically a lifestyle issue.

Just as many waking life problems are rooted in our sleep, most sleep problems are rooted in our waking lives. They are typically associated with an array of health, psychological, and environmental factors, most of which are linked to lifestyle. Lifestyle issues cannot be fixed with simple pills or potions, tricks or tweaks. More often than not, what we must do to heal our sleep is precisely what we must do to heal our waking lives.

ᘒ18ᘓ

Count your blessings instead
of counting sheep.

Thinking about the good things we already have, helps shift
our attention away from the anxious provocation of needs,
wants, and desires. Gratitude is an exceptional sleep elixir. It's
a natural sedative that calms the mind and soothes the spirit
with absolutely no side effects. Make a list of things you are
grateful for tonight and slip it under your pillow. Plan to add a
good night's sleep to your list upon awakening.

ᴄ❩ 19 ᴄ❩

**If awakening is a kind of rebirth,
then early morning is the childhood
of the rest of our day.**

We awaken each morning from dreams that have helped us
digest and assimilate yesterday's experiences. We awaken
renewed. And as we come to, we have an opportunity to
mindfully establish a trajectory for our new day. Guide yourself
upon awakening as you would lovingly guide a child -- not with
complex instructions about activity, but with simple notions
about attitude. The attitudes we establish upon awakening will
powerfully imbue their qualities into the rest of our day.

∽20∾

Because many of us abruptly awaken at night not from sleep but from dreams, it's essential to establish a dialog with them.

In 'To sleep per chance to dream…' Hamlet voices a most common reason we resist sleep -- anxiety about the challenging dreams that it might bring. Clearly evident in posttraumatic nightmares, the fear of recurring dark dreams can readily result in sleeplessness. For most of us, premature morning awakenings suggest the possibility that we are avoiding our dreams. Dreams are healing. Consider a rapprochement with them. Explore dreamwork to open a dialog with and even befriend your dreams.

∽ 21 ∼

Where do we go when we go to sleep?

If water is a universal symbol of the unconscious, sleep is the liquid substrate of our lives. We can sink into it, yet it supports us. Just as when we were in the womb, we are spiritually amphibious in the sea of sleep. But our willingness to descend into the depths of these waters depends on what we believe we might actually encounter there. Nothing? Nightmares? Restoration? Dreams? Serenity? Intentionally descending into the sea of sleep with our inner, 'third eye' open can help us reflect on this key question.

∽22∾

Middle of the night wakefulness was once understood to be a normal and natural feature of sleep.

Substantial evidence from historical research suggests that prior to the industrial revolution, people routinely awakened in the middle of the night for an hour or two. This period of "night watch" was a special time during which people would socialize, pray, make love, or reflect on their dreams -- in the deep stillness of candlelit nights. Consider adopting a nightwatch approach instead greeting middle of the night awakenings with an expletive.

∽23∾

To descend deeply into the sweet waters of sleep, we must stop focusing on the shoreline of tomorrow morning's awakening.

When the lights go out and we slip into bed and close our eyes, where does our attention go? Too often our thoughts are not so much about surrendering to sleep, but rather about dashing through sleep to get to the next morning's awakening. "What will I wear tomorrow? What's available for breakfast? How will I manage the day?" Are we reflexively fixating on the shoreline of tomorrow morning's awakening, or will we allow ourselves to descend deeply into the sea of sleep?

᧐24᧐

Waking and dreaming are made of the same fluid consciousness.

The word consciousness has no plural. Waking is a form of dreaming and dreaming is a kind of waking. Both are expressions of the very same watery awareness as it streams through different landscapes. Waking is like a river whose depth and flow is defined and directed by the earthy banks that give it shape and form. Dreaming is the open and expansive deep sea of experience into which this river of waking empties. It should not be a surprise that our dream and waking lives have so much in common.

❧25❧

Morning grogginess is an exquisite state of mind.

We do not typically awaken directly from sleep, but rather from our dreams. In striking contrast to its derivation from the English rum drink, grog, the term "grogginess" actually refers to an exquisite, hybrid state of sleep, dreams, and waking. If we refrain from dismissing it or yanking ourselves out of it, grogginess offers us a glimpse into a beautiful, fluid, and unified experience of consciousness.

∽26∾

The number of hours we spend asleep is no better a measure of healthy slumber than the number of calories we eat is of healthy nutrition.

Preoccupation with the quantity of our sleep distracts us from the more pertinent question about the quality of our sleep. Just as focusing on caloric intake tells us nothing about the nutrients we are consuming, our total sleep time tells us nothing about the quality of our sleep or the quality of our dreaming. The best measure of healthy sleep is healthy waking -- a natural ebb and flow of vitality, relaxation, creativity and good spirits.

∽27∾

Scaring ourselves about the dire consequences of sleep loss will not help us regain our sleep.

Although it might seem like a reasonable way of motivating sleep improvement, ruminating about the negative health ramifications of sleep loss when we can't sleep will only exacerbate our sleeplessness. It's true that chronic sleep loss can compromise our health in the long term. But humans are particularly resilient creatures. If we don't sleep well tonight, it doesn't mean we'll awaken with a terrible illness tomorrow.

$\backsim$28$\backsim$

Going to sleep without ritual is like making love without foreplay.

Approaching sleep in a mechanistic way will only dampen its pleasure. It's especially helpful to be mindful of our love of sleep before going to bed. There is no better way of doing this than by establishing a personal pre-sleep ritual. Ordinary bedtime routines can readily be transformed into enjoyable bedtime rituals simply by enacting them mindfully -- by imbuing a sense of meaning into them. Bedtime rituals that directly support our release of waking are particularly conducive to pleasurable sleep.

∽ 29 ∾

We are at least as dream deprived as we are sleep deprived.

Many aspects of modern lifestyles interfere with REM sleep and healthy dreaming. Numerous commonly used medications as well as alcohol and substances can suppress dreaming. Virtually all antidepressants and anti-anxiety medications compromise our dreams. Excessive exposure to light at night as well as early morning sleeplessness and sleep apnea also tamp down our dreams. The widespread, chronic loss of dreaming is an unrecognized public and spiritual health hazard that is silently wreaking havoc with our lives.

⌒30⌒

Sleep is the internal representation of night.

Night is not simply an environmental state; it's also an internal psychological and spiritual experience. If we allow it, the sun will also set within us, our energy will wane, and we will become nocturnal. Like an owl in the dark wood, sleep naturally comes to life under the cover of night.

∽ 31 ∾

Sleep is not a respite from life, but a deeper immersion into it.

Too often, we think of sleep as time subtracted from life. But this is only the case if we limit our definition of life to include only the waking hours. Hugh Prather taught that *life is lived in the pauses, not the events.* Sleep is certainly among the most poignant of such pauses. The incomparable respite and rejuvenation offered us in sleep is not a subtraction from but is an enhancement of life.

༄32ༀ

How we react to sleepiness by day will impact how sleepiness will respond to us at night.

Daytime sleepiness is about sleep, a welcomed guest at night, arriving at an inopportune time. When we habitually go to battle with daytime somnolence, our relationship with nighttime sleep becomes negatively conditioned. Our guest may become skittish or wary of us at bedtime. Forgive and make peace with daytime sleepiness. Negotiate with it. Give it a little kind attention now with the promise of much more receptivity later.

33

Sleep is grace.

Like gravity, sleep is invisible, omnipresent, and gently but persistently grounding. Like the sandman sprinkling sleepy dust over the eyes of children, sleep is a gift that is sprinkled graciously from above. If we are receptive -- if we are simply open to receiving it -- sleep will gently usher us back to a place of rest, rejuvenation, healing, and serenity. But we must be willing to receive it as a gift.

↶34↷

"Lose your dreams and you will lose your mind." -- Mick Jagger

Psychologists have long characterized depression as a loss of one's dreams. The nightly dreaming pattern most commonly seen in depressed individuals is strikingly similar to those of research subjects who have had their dreaming suppressed. With the chronic devaluation and loss of our dreams, the color is slowly bleached from our lives and we experience depression -- waking life devoid of its naturally expansive and mysterious context. It would make sense then that healing depression would call for a restoration of healthy dreaming.

∽35∽

If we routinely awaken with an alarm clock, we are never getting enough sleep.

It's been said there is no hope for a civilization that starts each day to the sound of an alarm. Though this may be overstated, the alarm clock is a ubiquitous symbol of our widespread devaluation of sleep. When we are awakened by an alarm clock, we snip off the end of our sleep and dreams. Would we consider setting a timer to artificially limit the time we spend at dinner or in lovemaking? Going to bed a little earlier each night until we are able to awaken naturally can help us break this habit.

∽36∾

Sleep and waking are not opposite or mutually exclusive experiences. They can and frequently do coexist.

When we are drifting into sleep or arising from it, some degree of waking is clearly present. When we are sleepy during the day or wakeful at night, we are also experiencing a mix of both sleep and waking consciousness. In fact, it may be that we are always to varying degrees both asleep and awake. It's interesting to notice the wispy presence of sleep even when we feel wide awake. And although more challenging, the presence of awareness even when we are asleep.

∽37∾

Women are generally much better and much worse sleepers than men.

Women are at greater risk for sleeplessness than men. The ebb and flow of hormones associated with menstruation, pregnancy and menopause leaves them more susceptible to sleep disruption. But women also appear to be biologically predisposed to get significantly more deep sleep than men. This may be Mother Nature's way of compensating for the special challenges associated with childbearing and motherhood.

❧38❧

The thinking part of us is simply incapable of accessing or delivering sleep.

As useful as thinking might be in waking life, it inhibits sleep just as light inhibits night. And just as we can walk along the water's edge, but cannot walk in deep water, we can think our way to the brink of slumber, but not directly into deeper sleep. Thinking can be useful in setting the stage for our surrender to sleep. But the actual transition into sleep requires willingness to let go of thinking. Think about it...

ᵔ39ᵔ

Bad dreams are like frightening movies; they are plentiful and unsettling yet intriguing.

What makes even the scariest movies tolerable is maintaining some degree of awareness that we are seated safely in a cinema or in our living rooms. Bad dreams and nightmares are normal, common and much easier to manage if we cultivate mindfulness of the fact that we are actually resting securely in the theater of our beds.

ᘒ40ᘓ

The bed stand clock tells us what time it is in the waking world. Why monitor the time in a place where we don't want to be?

When we can't sleep and a clock is nearby, it's nearly impossible to resist the temptation to check the time. But doing so only yanks us back into our waking world ways. Many of us then do the math, calculating how much sleep we might get if we could just nod out again soon. This only further tethers us to wakefulness. Most digital bed stand clocks also emit a lot of light, which suppresses melatonin and compromises our sleep as well as our long-term health. Clocks should stay in the waking world.

∽ 41 ∾

We can never fully understand sleep from a waking world frame of mind.

Viewing sleep solely through our waking world eyes is like trying to observe darkness by using a flashlight. Sleep is best understood by deluminating it, both literally and figuratively. In giving our waking world senses a rest, we step into a nighttime frame of mind or night consciousness. In this shadowy world, we encounter sleep in its natural home.

∽42∾

Sometimes we are reluctant to let go of this day simply because we don't want to face the next one.

The anticipation of awakening to a new day brimming with demands and expectations can effectively deter us from sleep. It may seem that the next day will arrive in a blink: I close my eyes and when I reopen them it's tomorrow. In reality, so much can be transformed in that blink. Our bodies, minds, and spirits are remade in sleep and dreams. Morning can look very different when night's eyes have had a chance to rest.

◌⃝43◌⃝

Rest is the natural bridge between waking and sleep.

Rest is too frequently confused with recreation and even inebriation. It is neither. Brainwave patterns associated with true rest are identical to those observed in the transition from waking to sleep. Just as we must learn to walk before we can run, we must learn to rest before we can sleep. Rest is a wakeful form of sleep.

༄44༅

We remember dreams in much the same way we remember waking experiences -- by paying attention to them.

Think, talk, write, and read about dreams. Ask others about their dreams and listen with the same interest you would have if these were waking life experiences. In fact, they can affect us in much the same way. Regularly sharing dreams with a friend or partner is an effective way to deepen intimacy. Although it's useful to consider the connections between our dream lives and our waking lives, this doesn't necessarily require any formal analysis.

⌒45⌒

**Our descent into the depths of sleep
by night supports our ascent toward
the heights of passion by day.**

Each day of our lives is a great circadian wave defined by a crest
of waking and a trough of sleep. The peaks of our daily waking
lives determine the gradients of our glide into the depths of
nightly rest and repose. And the rejuvenation we obtain there
provides the energy essential to launch us back to vibrant
waking. Consider getting off the bullet train of culture to ride
this great circadian wave of nature.

ᘯ46ᕀ

We need never sleep alone.

We tend to view sleep as a discretely solo experience --
something we do independently of the world around us. But
going to sleep alone doesn't mean we'll be alone when we arrive
there. The experience of sleep doesn't segregate us from life;
it delivers us to an expansive shared world of dreams. From a
global perspective, dreaming can be viewed as a social event.
We sleep locally, dream globally.

∽47∾

Although we might feel terribly alone in our sleeplessness, in reality, the night is crowded with insomniacs.

Sleeplessness is often associated with a sense of isolation and loneliness. We are reluctant to wake our partner or call a friend. If we broaden our perspective, however, we realize that we're not alone. Our neighborhood, our community, indeed, our world inevitably includes so many others struggling in the very same way. Tens of millions of us experience sleeplessness on a nightly basis. It may be helpful to think about others nearby who might also be awake and believing they are alone.

$\sim$48$\sim$

To fall asleep peacefully, we must be willing to spend some time alone with ourselves --- in the dark.

It normally takes ten to twenty minutes or so to cross the border from waking into sleep. For too many of us, those moments between lights out and nodding out are the only opportunity we have to be fully present with ourselves. Often we are uncomfortable spending such undistracted time alone because it brings us face to face with thoughts and feelings that we have suppressed by day. Taking some time to be fully present with ourselves during waking hours is essential for an easier transition to sleep.

☌49☍

Dreaming is waking liberated from the constraints of the physical body.

During REM sleep, the river of waking consciousness widens into the sea of sleep and dreams. We become "disembodied," that is, able to experience life independently of any sensations or activities in the world. Spiritual perspectives commonly view this process in terms of the soul leaving the body. When the flow of consciousness is no longer framed, constrained and grounded by the body's sensory or motor experience, it is free to become transcendent and magical.

༄50༄

Two sleepers in one bed can be like two sides of one beating heart.

Most couples spend the bulk of their together time asleep bed. Despite this, the night side of relationship is rarely considered and the number of couples sleeping apart is now increasing dramatically. Sharing sleep is much like sharing a meal or a walk. Sleeping together can help synchronize our circadian rhythms, enhance empathy, and promote shared awakenings. Recognize it as time spent together. Think of it as a very long, very slow dance.

ᘓ 51 ᘔ

Sleep is literally cool and dreaming is the coolest part of night.

Just like the outside world when the sun goes down, our body temperature naturally drops when we go down. We are designed to release heat -- to dissipate energy throughout the night. And we reach our coolest point near dawn, during our most protracted period of dreams. Overactivity, overeating, and overthinking can contribute to our overheating. Chill out in the evening. Sleeping in a cool bedroom will also help us stay cool.

⌒52⌒

For better sleep we must balance 'taking something to sleep' with 'letting go of something to sleep.'

There are two fundamental approaches to managing sleeplessness: taking something to sleep and letting go of something to sleep. Whether they are dietary supplements, sleeping pills, warm milk or bedtime snacks, taking something to promote sleep typically increases our sleepiness. But it does nothing to quell the noise within us. Letting go of something to sleep is about identifying and quieting this noise. Taking something to sleep works best when complemented with letting go of something to sleep.

⌒53⌒

We don't have to turn off our mental radio to get to sleep, but we do need to lower the volume and stop listening to it.

Our thoughts can seem so much larger, louder, and more compelling against the backdrop of night. No longer tempered by the competing stimulation of the waking world, thoughts can easily dominate consciousness at that time, obscuring the more subtle call of sleep. To tune out our thoughts, we must first ask ourselves what we believe is of greater value -- our inner talk radio show or a good night's sleep. Then we can practice simply shifting our attention from the waking mind to our sleepy body.

∽54∾

Write about your day as if it were a dream.

A daily journal or diary can help us observe and appreciate the larger story of our lives. Writing about our daily lives as if they were dreams can do the same for the deeper back-story of our lives. Simply think about your day as if it were a dream. Review it through dream eyes, noticing dream-like images, experiences, and themes.

55

Napping is seditious and subversive. Do it.

We typically think of rebellious or unruly behavior in terms of disobedient action. But given our culture's overvaluing stance toward activity and productivity along with its judgmental posture toward rest and sleep, napping is one of the simplest and certainly most enjoyable ways to protest. Naps are a rejuvenating coup against common culture's insane pace.

$\backsim56\backsim$

Sooner or later, we must come to terms with the uneasy kinship of sleep and death.

The association of sleep and death is acknowledged in many sacred traditions around the world. Hypnos, the Greek god of sleep, was brother to Thanatos, the god of death. The Talmud suggests that sleep is made up of a small part of death. Tibetan Buddhism teaches that the psychospiritual process of falling asleep parallels that of dying. It's not a surprise that the classic Christian bedtime prayer, "…if I die before I awake, I pray the Lord my soul to take," has left many a child sharply ambivalent about sleep. Sleep and death require a similar kind of surrender. But in reality, the vast majority of us do not die in our sleep, but rather, we pass on during waking. (Yet another reason to sleep more.)

৵57৵

The simplest yet most challenging aspect of getting to sleep is the surrender of our relentless effort.

Sleeplessness is commonly linked to excessive sleep effort. That is, we try too hard to get to sleep. Trying too hard to not try too hard is the very same mistake in a different form. To give up effort is to surrender. It's in this willingness to lose the battle that we let go of waking. Falling asleep is not something we need to control or direct. It's a ride and we are just passengers.

⌒58⌒

Our descent through night and touchdown into sleep frequently involves negotiating a layer of personal turbulence.

Jet planes usually cruise above the weather and then typically descend through some turbulence to land. Likewise, many of us soar above our emotions throughout our busy waking days and then encounter psychological turbulence when slowing to land at night. Because bumpy updrafts of unresolved feelings can make it challenging to slow, land and come to a full stop, it's best to fully descend before touching down in bed.

⌒⤳**59**⤳⌐

Even very bad dreams can be an expression of a good dream life.

Challenging dreams are as common as challenges in waking life. And just as difficult life events can promote personal growth, so it is with difficult dreams. The characteristic postures we assume toward challenges are strikingly parallel in both worlds. In dreams, however, we are free to practice new and creative ways of being -- to exercise courage with great impunity.

⌒60⌒

Ordinary clock time is much too dynamic to accommodate sleep.

To sleep well, we need to reconsider our understanding of time. There are, in fact, two different types of time -- day and night time. Day or ordinary clock time is linear, progressive, and relentless. It streams nonstop from the past through the present and on into the future. It's defined by continually changing numbers that never slow, let alone stop. It never sleeps.

61

It's best to acknowledge our love of sleep before we slip into bed with it.

Truly good sleepers will sometimes confess that they "love sleep." That they "*really* love sleep." And they mean it. Somewhere earlier in our lives, most of us had a subconscious love affair with sleep. But for too many, the relentless distraction of waking life has compromised this relationship. To fall back in love with sleep we must begin by acknowledging its beauty and conscientiously courting it.

⌒62⌒

What kinds of emotions do we bring to bed with us at night? Can we sleep comfortably along side of them?

Some emotions are a pleasure to sleep with, some not so pleasant but still cooperative, and others can make sleep difficult, if not impossible. Contentment, joy, hope and affection are easy. Although considered negative emotions, sadness, sorrow and loneliness are quiet and will not necessarily interfere with sleep. In contrast, restless emotions like anxiety, fear, anger and resentment can toss, turn, kick, and poke at us throughout the night. It may be helpful to strike a deal with such feelings, asking them to wait outside of the bedroom until morning when you'll willingly attend to them.

ᴄ᷾᷉63ᴄᷧ

Although it can be both addictive and contagious, laughter is an exceptional sleep elixir.

Laughter quells the body, quiets the mind and soothes the spirit. Whether through watching a sitcom, reading something lighthearted or engaging in a friendly tickle fight, intentionally eliciting a good belly laugh or two before bed is an excellent means of loosening our grip on the day and preparing for sweet slumber. Whatever might stand between you and that nightly last laugh is likely what is standing between you and good sleep.

༄64༄

Dreams are a secret garden
hidden in plain view.

Even if we cannot see dreams with our waking world eyes, we can detect their subtle fragrance as night blooms at the edge of twilight. Dreaming is the star field that encompasses the entire world. It's the very ground that the house of wakefulness is built upon. All we need do is peek out the window of waking with our dream eyes to witness this more numinous world.

∽65∾

The best strategy in our war against sleeplessness is surrender.

We wage war against illness. We fight disease, kill germs, and go to battle with our symptoms. This is most evident with insomnia. Many of us silently hurl expletives at our nighttime wakefulness. But the peace of sleep cannot be realized through an inner civil war. To sleep well, we must learn to approach sleep in a thoroughly nonviolent way. Giving up this fight is not about a forced supplication, but rather, a gracious surrender.

⌒66⌒

Sleep is another world.

In sleep we enter a fundamentally different kind of
consciousness -- another place and another kind of time. We're
not in Kansas anymore. Thinking about sleep while awake is
like peering across the border into a foreign land. It's a strange
yet strikingly familiar culture that can only be understood and
accepted on its own terms. We might think of the bedroom as a
border town.

∽ 67 ∾

If, as the Bible says, "God gives sleep to those He loves," what does that imply about insomniacs?

Even if we do not agree with this notion, too many of us harbor a subtle sense of guilt when we can't sleep. We rack our brains and search our souls for the mistakes we may have made that led to our sleeplessness. Frequently, however, the major mistake is the subtle undercurrent of self-blame that fuels these thoughts. Forgiveness is a great sleep elixir, an essential foundation for healing our sleep. Begin by forgiving yourself and then forgive your sleeplessness.

ꙮ68ꙮ

There is nothing that we have to do to get to sleep, but we must be willing to do that.

We toss and turn, get up and go back down, get a drink, and then empty our bladders. We might pray or meditate or just think hard about not thinking. Maybe we mull over all the possible causes of our sleeplessness, taking time to chastise ourselves for that late caffeinated beverage. We may agonize over not being able stop our minds from thinking relentlessly about why they are thinking so relentlessly. We cannot get to sleep through intention, exertion, or effort.

↶ 69 ↷

Dreaming is not just something we passively experience; it reflects our personal posture toward all experience.

Our dreams offer ongoing reflections of how we respond to a vast array of experiences from the ordinary and mundane to the mythic and fantastic. Dreams provide irrefutable evidence of our greatest fears and our deepest faith. Dreaming reflects the extent of our willingness to relate to the unknown. In dreams, we are offered opportunities to experiment and experience anything and everything without disturbing the waking world.

ᴄ70ᴄ

Night is another kind of time.

Night is usually seen as a subset of day. But what we call nighttime is not just a part of day's time. Nighttime, or more accurately, night's time, does not go anywhere. It's comforting, receptive, and rhythmic, revolving around a center point of stillness. It's naturally sedating, gently rocking and lulling us into slumber. Night's time is a wheel with sleep as its timeless hub. When we fall asleep, we tumble out of time.

∽ 71 ∽

The bedroom is a temple -- a personal sanctuary and portal to night consciousness.

We frequently smuggle a waking world mindset into our bedrooms at night. Consequently, the modern bedroom has evolved into an entertainment center that keeps us tethered to the waking world. An optimal bedroom is like a temple -- a liminal space entered into through ritual. It serves as both a sanctuary from waking life and a portal to the ethereal consciousness of sleep and dreams. It's a good place to pray, meditate and, of course, dream.

$\backsim$72$\backsim$

Too much wakeful time spent in bed can cause accidental sleeplessness.

Just as it's critical to avoid driving when we are sleepy, it's important to stay out of bed when we are persistently wakeful. If we have a history of insomnia, it's helpful to get into bed only when we feel sleepy. And to get out of bed to relax or meditate when we are wakeful until we feel drowsy. Just as we want to associate our car with alertness, we want to associate our bed with drowsiness.

✑73✑

Going out like a light when your head hits the pillow is not a sign of being a good sleeper.

Although my mother might have thought differently, quickly scarfing down one's lunch is not a sign of being a good eater. It might, in fact, suggest that one is excessively hungry. Since it's normal to take about twenty minutes to drift into sleep, a routine pattern of rapid sleep onset is suggestive of being excessively sleepy, which may be the result of an underlying sleep problem.

↶74↷

Capture, coddle and carry your dreams into the waking world.

Leaving our dreams in bed and under cover by day reinforces the illusion of segregated consciousness -- of the separate worlds of night and day. By carefully attending to, journaling or talking about our dreams, we bring that innocent and expansive way of perceiving into the waking world. Viewing waking life through dream eyes helps restore mystery and meaning as well as a sense of the continuity of consciousness.

∽75∾

Cultivating a personal sense of deep safety is essential for deep sleep.

In sleep, we are all vulnerable to both the world around us as well as the world within us. Freely surrendering to sleep requires feeling perfectly safe from any external intrusions. Such safety is as much a personal as it is a rational matter. We must also cultivate a sense of security in the world of sleep and dreams. It's useful to ask ourselves what exactly might offer us such safety and security and to do all it takes to obtain them.

∼76∼

We can practice keeping sleep close at hand even throughout our waking day.

"Sleep lingers all our lifetime about our eyes, as night hovers all day in the boughs of the fir-tree," wrote Ralph Waldo Emerson. Keeping sleep close by during our waking hours makes it much easier to return to it at night. This is most evident in cats and dogs, who are usually able to slip into sleep whenever the opportunity arises. We can, upon awakening, choose to gather and carry the stillness of sleep and the enchantment of dreams with us like a talisman throughout the day.

⌒77⌒

Gravity is the covert manifestation
of sleep in the waking world.

There is an aspect of the environment that is always asleep.
Gravity watches over us constantly and literally keeps us
grounded. We are rarely aware of it until we witness it in action
behind a fall. We can experience gravity most clearly when we
let go. Letting ourselves fall under the spell of gravity is a most
effective way to transition to sleep. Tune into it. Get into bed
with it. Feel it gently but firmly against your body.

⌒78⌒

Consider flirting with sleepiness
before getting into bed with it.

Just as we can more readily sense gravity when we push against it, sleep becomes more palpable when we momentarily resist it. Feel around for and gently lean into your sleepiness. Press against it and sense its soft but firm push back. Let it meet and embrace you like a caring and cuddly friend. Playfully resist the growing heaviness in your eyelids and your head. And then just let go.

⌒79⌒

Examining a dream with our waking world eyes is like looking at the night sky through sunglasses.

Dreams are intriguing. But we typically proceed to interpret them without first addressing the more basic question of what dreaming is. This is like trying to interpret a painting without understanding what art is. Just as it makes no sense to examine a work of art in terms of its utility, so do our dreams become distorted and misinterpreted when viewed solely through our utilitarian waking world lenses. Sadly, this is precisely what most popular approaches to dream interpretation do.

⌒⌒80⌒⌒

Overstressing our desire to be awake throughout the day can override our ability to sleep at bedtime.

It's helpful to become aware of the extent of energy and intention we invest in promoting wakefulness throughout our day. Relentlessly pressuring ourselves to be focused, productive, functional, and efficient creates a momentum that can be difficult to tame at night. Taking periodic rest breaks to remember and touch into the presence of sleep will help us modulate our attachment to waking.

ᘓ 81 ᘒ

Stories are the royal road to sleep. What's your story?

Virtually all cultures engage in nightly story telling. Whether they are grand myths about the collective unconscious, tales about ordinary life, or classic childhood bedtime stories, they guide us in understanding our personal experiences. We all live out the stories of our lives one day at a time. Reviewing these stories in the evening is one of the best ways of processing and letting go of the day to surrender to night and sleep.

ꞈ82ꞈ

Just as a good day does not guarantee
a good night, a bad night does not
inevitably lead to a bad day.

Our certainty that a night of poor sleep will ruin the next day
can heighten anxiety, which further compromises our sleep
and the quality of the following day. Whatever else humans
might be, we are also remarkably resilient. In reality, our
daytime energy naturally ebbs and flows and doesn't depend
exclusively on the amount of sleep we obtained the night
before. We will better manage the next day if we relinquish
our anxiety about it.

∾83∾

Crying oneself to sleep is not an illegitimate way of getting there.

Sadness, sorrow, and grief are not uncommon visitors to our waking lives. Contrary to what many of us believe, we don't need to fully process (or suppress) these emotions before we can sleep. In fact, we need to sleep and dream well before we can thoroughly heal through them. Unlike resentment or anxiety, we can sleep alongside the stillness of loss and grief.

∽84∾

More important than knowing the meaning of any particular dream is knowing that dreaming is meaningful.

Most approaches to dream analysis or interpretation try to help us make psychological sense of a dream by explaining it in terms of waking life. Ultimately, we will get that dreams are meaningful not through interpretation or analysis, but simply by experiencing them. To do this, we need first to stop dismissing our dreams. And then we need to stop coming at them with preconceived waking world notions.

〜85〜

Our inner clock does not keep time; it maintains a sense of timing.

Our inner clock doesn't know what day of the week it is, only that it is day or night. It doesn't know what month it is, but it can sense the season. It doesn't know what year it is and it doesn't really care. Our inner clock doesn't keep ordinary time but instead operates on cyclic or rhythmic timing. We can look to clocks to tell us what time it is. But we must look inside to tune into the sense of timing that governs our sleep and dreams.

∽86∾

Struggles with accessing deeper sleep are struggles with accessing deeper parts of ourselves.

How much of who we believe we are is limited to our waking world identity? Are there parts of ourselves that become more visible in the dark -- in the deeper waters of sleep and dreams? Deep sleep can help deliver us to these veiled, unconscious aspects of our selves. Whatever might stand between us and deep sleep also stands between us and our deeper selves.

ᦓ87ᦓ

It's best to descend gradually into sleep like the sun into the sea.

We cannot dive directly into the depths of the sea of sleep at the shoreline of waking. Because the waters here are shallow, we run the risk of hitting the ground of wakefulness. We need instead to be patient and gradually wade into the depths. We need to practice a slower immersion in which we willingly offer ourselves up, little by little, to these mysterious waters.

ᴄ⌒88⌒ᴄ

What wakes us up at night is not what typically keeps us up.

Any number of psychological, medical or environmental factors can draw us back to the waking world from sleep. We may be aware of these, as is common, for example, with the need to use the bathroom. More often we are unaware of exactly what rouses us. It might be subtle symptoms of indigestion, the start of a provocative dream, or ambient light. Whatever the cause, we generally assume that what woke us up is also what is keeping us awake. In fact, what typically perpetuates our wakefulness is not what woke us up but our cognitive reaction to it.

↷89↶

It's not about conjuring conviction in our ability to sleep, but about cultivating willingness to get out of sleep's way.

Many of us lose faith in our very capacity to sleep. With ongoing struggles we come to doubt ourselves and believe that we somehow need to rebuild confidence in our ability to get to sleep. This is the waking part of us thinking it can strategize its way back to sleep when, in fact, it has never been there. Falling asleep is not an act of volition. We cannot literally go to sleep. But we can become willing to let go of waking.

⌒90⌒

How can we teach our children to sleep well? Through simple demonstration.

Children learn more from what they observe than from what they are told. They learn basic lessons about sleep from observing their parents, family and caregivers. When they see adults valuing and enjoying sleep, they will open to similar experiences. When they see adults resisting sleep and overvaluing waking, they will be inclined to do the same. The converse is also true: adults can be reminded of sleep's true nature by taking a few moments to just watch children in sweet slumber.

ᓚ 91 ᓗ

Falling asleep is like falling in love. Both call for willingness to surrender.

Whether at the start or in the middle of the night, falling asleep is not an act of will but rather one of willingness. Surrender, a sweet and trusting relinquishment of will, should not be confused with supplication, a sense of forced submission to something we don't want. When slipping into bed, make the surrender of your waking self more important than submission to sleep.

༄92༄

Desperately seeking sleep will only bring us desperation, not sleep.

The attitudes underlying our strategies for getting to sleep are at least as important as the strategies themselves. It's fine to make a gentle effort to surrender waking. But if we are doing even the most helpful things in desperation, they will fail to facilitate sleep. The means by which we approach sleep will define the quality of our sleep -- or sleeplessness.

ᘒ93ᘗ

Healing our sleep requires more than change in behaviors; it calls for a change of heart.

Tips for obtaining better sleep abound. But the common presumption that we can simply tinker and tweak our way to good sleep is misguided. Sleep tips work best in the context of a personal sleep transformation. Healthy sleep requires a shift in our fundamental perspective and basic attitudes. It requires a willingness to meet sleep on its own otherworldly terms.

ᐫ94ᐭ

Napping is an excellent alternative to nibbling.

Since hunger and sleepiness are both low energy states, the two can be easily confused. Taking a moment to be mindful of what we really need and then conjuring the compassion to offer it to ourselves will improve both our sleep and waking lives. Brief midday naps are refreshing for the body, mind and spirit.

∽95∾

We dream all the time.

We believe we dream only at night for the same reason we believe stars come out only at night. Although dreaming is most evident when seen through the windows of nightly REM sleep, it's always present. When we no longer see dreaming as the exclusive province of night, when we intentionally carry elements of the dream into the waking world, we open our hearts to the re-enchantment of daily life.

⌒96⌒

We can approach sleep as a sacred ritual -- a spiritual practice.

If "Sleep is the best meditation," as the Dalai Lama says, then consider what an additional 7 or 8 hours of daily spiritual practice might mean in your life. We can cultivate a gentle mindfulness around our sleep process, but we do not need to be awake in the ordinary sense to witness our sleep and dreams. We need only consider that there is something there worth experiencing. In deep sleep we are graciously granted admission to the place accomplished spiritual practitioners journey. Sleep is the lazy aspirant's path to serenity.

ᕲ97ᕷ

The bridge to sleep can safely carry us over troubled waters.

Are we required to address our major problems as a prerequisite to surrendering to sleep? Actually, it's possible to sleep quite well with pressing relationship issues, alongside of illness, and even while knowing that there are dirty dinner dishes in the sink. In fact, good sleep is a prerequisite to the effective resolution of all such problems.

∽98∽

If we knew with certainty that life is but a dream, we would live with the promise of a greater awakening.

In the Bible's creation story, Adam was not put into a deep sleep, but more of a deep dream. Nowhere in the remainder of Genesis, however, does God ever bother to awaken him. Because we ultimately awaken from our dreams, the practice of viewing ordinary daily life as a dream can help us cultivate a palpable faith in an eventual greater awakening.

⌒⌒99⌒⌒

Sleeplessness is a lesson in forgiveness.

At its root, the term "to forgive" means to "let go" or "give
back." Our fundamental challenge in getting to sleep is to let go
of waking -- to give it back. Our willingness to forgive waking,
to forgive the whole waking world, and to forgive our waking
sense of self is the key to healthy sleep. Good sleepers do this
instinctively. Those of us who are challenged with sleep issues
must learn to do this more mindfully.

❧100❧

The segregation of waking from sleep and dreams obscures the underlying unity of consciousness.

Just as the three primary colors can be mixed in various proportions to create an infinite array of hues, so the three primary forms of consciousness -- sleep, dreams and waking -- blend to create the boundless spectrum of human experience. The segregation of waking consciousness from sleep and dreams bifurcates our perception, reinforcing the delusion of living in a world of duality.

Dr. Rubin Naiman

Rubin Naiman, PhD is the sleep and dream specialist and clinical assistant professor of medicine at the world-renowned University of Arizona Center for Integrative Medicine, directed by Dr. Andrew Weil. He is founder and director of Circadian Health Associates, an organization that offers a broad range of sleep related services, training and consultation internationally.

Dr. Naiman is a leader in the development of integrative medicine approaches to sleep and dreams, creatively weaving medical perspectives with depth psychological and transpersonal views. He founded the sleep and dream programs at Canyon Ranch and Miraval Resorts and has served as the director of the Sleep and Dream Advisory Board for Sleep Studio. Dr. Naiman maintains a private practice in Tucson and has worked with a diverse clientele ranging from CEOs to world-class athletes and from homemakers to statesmen and entertainers.

Dr. Naiman is the author of a number of groundbreaking works on sleep and dreams, including:

- Healing Night: The Science and Spirit of Sleeping, Dreaming, and Awakening
- Healthy Sleep (with Andrew Weil, MD)
- The Yoga of Sleep: Sacred and Scientific Practices to Heal Sleeplessness
- To Sleep Tonight

He also blogs about sleep and dreams for the Huffington Post and Psychology Today. Dr. Naiman's website is www.drnaiman.com.

CPSIA information can be obtained
at www.ICGtesting.com
Printed in the USA
LVOW12s1541011017
550765LV00003B/570/P